Easy Carnivore Diet on A Budget

The Beginner's Guide to Carnivore Diet, How to Start, What to Eat, And How to Enjoy Your Meal-Based Carnivore Diet for Weight Loss Without Hurting Your Pocket.

Gladys Wealth

Contents

INTRODUCTION

One major reason why people do not engage in the carnivore diet is because they believe it's quite expensive and a diet that is only befitting for kings.

What you should know is that the size of your bank account does not matter.

You don't necessarily have to be a member of the Rockefeller family before you can do this diet. Rather, you will be saving a whole lot of money by engaging in the carnivore diet.

If you are a beginner to the Carnivore diet, then this guide is for you. In it you will get exposed to tips on how to start, what to eat, and how do the diet without spending so much (cracking the edge), and so much more.

Just follow the steps explained in this guide and you can do the carnivore diet on a budget.

Tips to Do the Carnivore Diet on a Budget

1. Calculate Your Existing Food Budget

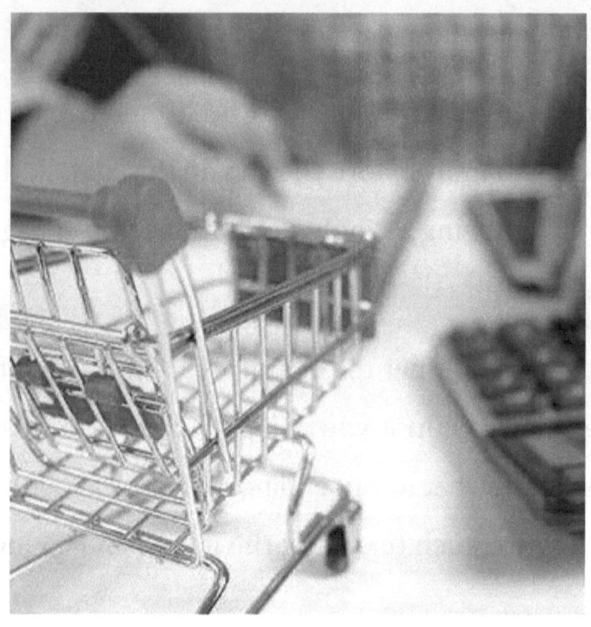

Before you step out to go and buy meat that will last up to three meals a day for the next week, you need to first determine how much you will spend on food.

What you need to do is to break it down into animal products and plants.

Now add up and get the total costs of all the non-dairy and non-meat stuff you buy.

You'll sure get surprised at how much it would be.

With this, you now know how much to aim for and try your best to get all your carnivore food planned out for the week within that total budget.

2. Work Out Your Exact Meat Intake

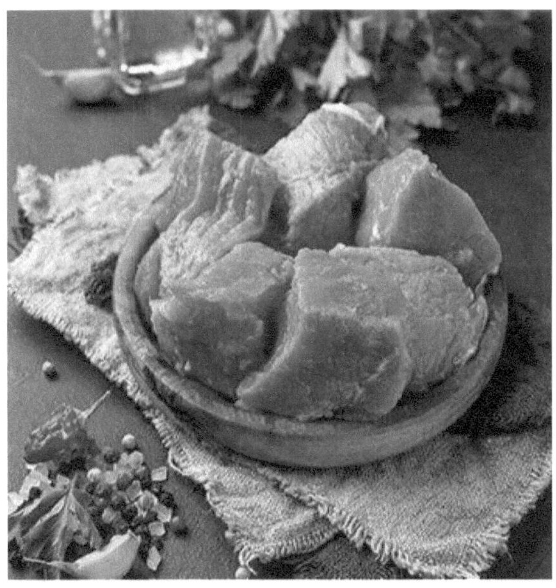

Keep in mind that you need an average energy need of 2,000 calories per day, so start creating a carnivore diet meal plan around that. But if you are a bodybuilder in a bulking phase, then you need to add about 10% or 20%, and if your goal is to shed some weight, then you should reduce it by at least 10%.

Note that the average cut of beef, chicken, and pork will contain about 600 calories per pound. But you can decide to stretch it from 600 to 800 calories by going for the cut with more fat.

You can also go for fat and oil-rich fish. It's a very good option and it can provide up to 1,000 calories per pound. And actually, you need up to 3 pounds of meat per day.

3. Get to know your local family butcher/find a local farm and buy in bulk.

As you now know the quantity of meat that you need each day, the next thing is to meet your local butcher and discuss with the owner about your meal plans. Also ask him directly if they can give you some reasonable prices as you will be buying in bulk on a weekly basis.

They will definitely welcome you with open arms and would also be willing to give you some advice on how to make your recipes a bit more varied.

The most common way to do the carnivore diet on a budget is to build a good relationship with a local farm and buy cuts in bulk from them. This way both of you can support a grass-fed ranch and eat conveniently on a budget.

Eat wild has helped to compile more than 1400 farms. It a may be a bit of an hassle going through the process as it is manual, but you can still make contact with farms around your locality and inquire about prices. If you place your order with a few friends, you might get an even bigger discount.

4. Buy/Experiment with Cheaper Cuts of Steak

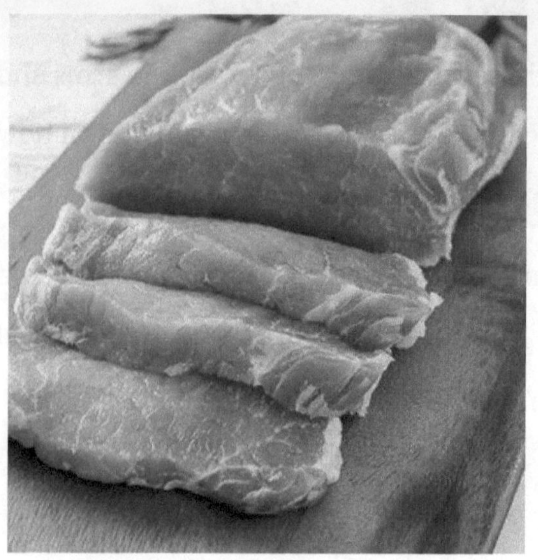

When you check for recipes online, you'll often see the top quality ingredients listed. Note that there are a lot of cuts of chicken, beef, pork, and even lamb that taste very good when prepared the right way.

You can get cheaper cuts of steak. You don't always have to eat a ribeye every day.

The cuts listed below are usually cheaper than the expensive ribeye's you often buy:

1.   Ground beef: the price for this is as low as $3.99 a pound. They are good for cheap and fatty meat, and since its ground, you don't have to cook it for too long.

2.   Chuck roast: A huge chunk of meat will cost about $3 or $4. You may need a crock pot to cook this.

3.   New York Strip: Sold for about $7 or $8 a lb

4.   Top Round

Going for these options can reduce costs drastically.

Given carnivores often eat less than 1 lb of meat per sitting, you'll be getting a full meal for less than $8 on the carnivore diet. It wouldn't be cheaper than that.

And the wonderful thing is that your butcher will be striving to sell them so that they can be bought very cheap.

Of course, they normally have more fat, but if you cook slowly the fat will just add up as a mouthwatering flavor.

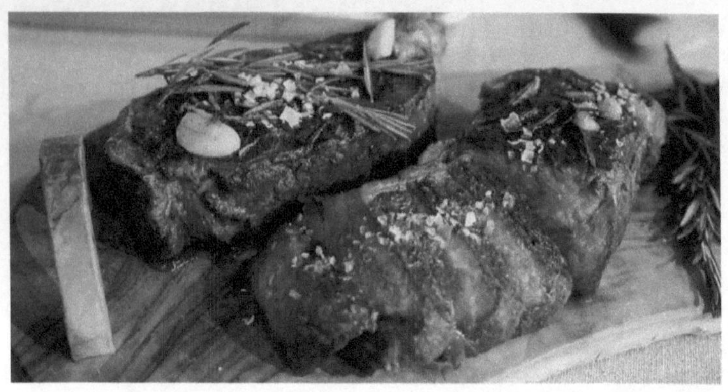

5. Opt for Grain Fed Instead of Grass Fed

When it comes to steak, quality matters a lot. If you can afford to pay up for a great grass-fed steak from a local, regenerative farm, I advise you do so.

However, you must not necessarily get your meat from a New Zealand farm where cows are hand massaged and sent to private school.

The truth is all meat is healthy — even from cows that don't eat the optimal diet.

The normal carnivore diet is way healthier than any other kind of diet, despite the quality of your food. The main nutrition equation is taking off all the crap in your existing diet.

In other words, don't allow perfect to become the enemy of good. Do your best to try out the carnivore diet, no matter the cost (but do not rob a bank!!)

Usually, grass-fed and organic beef do cost much more, majorly because they occupy more space and live longer.

You would possibly find grass-fed beef that's slightly close to grain-fed in price — especially when you buy in bulk — but on the average the price may be about 50% to 100% more.

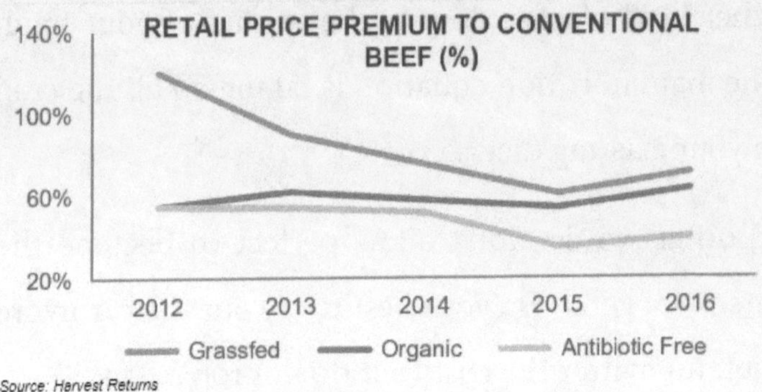

Research has shown that grass-fed beef has higher levels of Vitamin E, beta carotene, vitamin C and vitamin K2 than grain-fed beef. However, the levels of these vitamins in both forms of beef pale in comparison to those of other animal proteins.

For instance, liver has 275 times more Vitamin A than steak. And grass-fed fats such as tallow and suet have more vitamin E than other sources of vitamins, while butter, liver, and ghee can provide more K2

Red meat, despite the feeding regimen is nutrient-dense. But grass-fed fat has higher nutrient concentration, while grain-fed beef could have more fat. And since fat stores many of these nutrients, this may make things even.

6. Eat lots of Eggs, Beef Liver & Sardines

The three of the most nutritious foods in the world are actually the least expensive.

Eggs are one of these three and it is an absolute nutritional superfood. They usually make up for the nutrients that is lacking in beef muscle meat such as vitamin A retinol, choline, b vitamins, vitamin K2, selenium and vitamin E.

They are not only nutritious, but they taste very good and are extremely cheap.

And liver can be described as eggs on steroids.

(100g)	Blueberries	Kale	Beef	Beef Liver
Calcium	6.0 mg	72 mg	11 mg	11 mg
Phosphorus	12 mg	28 mg	140 mg	476 mg
Potassium	77 mg	228 mg	370 mg	380 mg
Iron	0.3 mg	0.9 mg	3.3 mg	8.8 mg
Zinc	0.2 mg	0.2 mg	4.4 mg	4.0 mg
Vitamin A	None	None	40 IU	53,400 IU
Vitamin D	None	None	Trace	19 IU
Vitamin E	0.6 mg	0.9 mg	1.7 mg	.63 mg
Vitamin C	9.7 mg	41 mg	None	27 mg
Niacin	0.4 mg	0.5 mg	4.0 mg	17 mg
Vitamin B6	0.1 mg	0.1 mg	.07 mg	.73 mg
Vitamin B12	None	None	1.8 mcg	111 mg
Folate	6 mcg	13 mcg	4.0 mcg	145 mcg

You will get 12 pasture raised eggs for about $6. You can also get 1 lb of grass-fed beef liver for $4 – $8.

Be aware that sardines and mackerel are not expensive at all, and they are also filled with nutrients like Vitamin B12, Vitamin D, selenium, bio-available DHA, and iodine. Wild planet sardines are sold for about $3.50 for 4 oz.

Eggs are a great source of protein, fat and cholesterol. And there are countless number of ways to prepare them

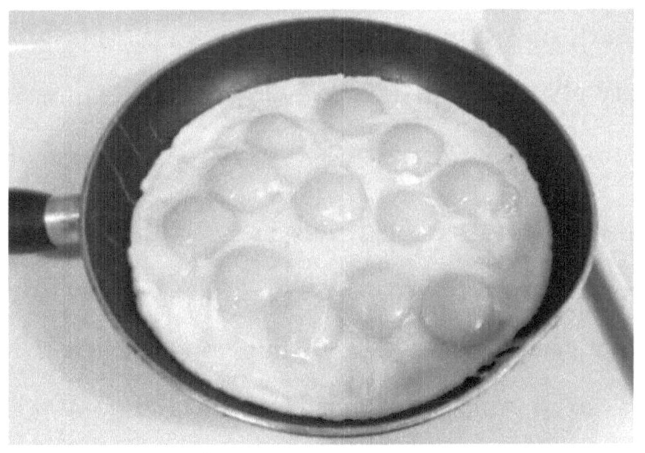

Eggs can be made as omelet, can be hard boiled, baked, poached, soft boil, scramble, sunny side up, over easy, over medium, over hard, basted, just name it.

7. Buy on Sale

In the days that we are now, brick and mortar retail is no longer in vogue especially with the rise of e-commerce. Consumers now have a more convenient time to do their grocery shopping, as these wearing-out retailers are doing everything possible to continue doing business in their stores. For example

Walmart, now offers free grocery pick up. And most grocery chains these days are also offering same, so go online and see what deals they have!

Mobile apps has made it easy now and Shipt and Instacart allows you to browse for grocery prices from all your stores nearby, with that you can compare prices, shop, and get it delivered all in the palm of your hand. The ability to do all of these while simply sitting on the couch is quite amazing!

Most grocery stores often run sales (weekly ad). Hopefully the world is going more vegan, so as a lover of meat you'll get more meat for yourself. But if you are interested in saving some money, start a no-beef challenge. Try out a week where you will possibly eat only chicken and pork. You can cut costs drastically by buying ground beef on sale in lieu of your steaks.

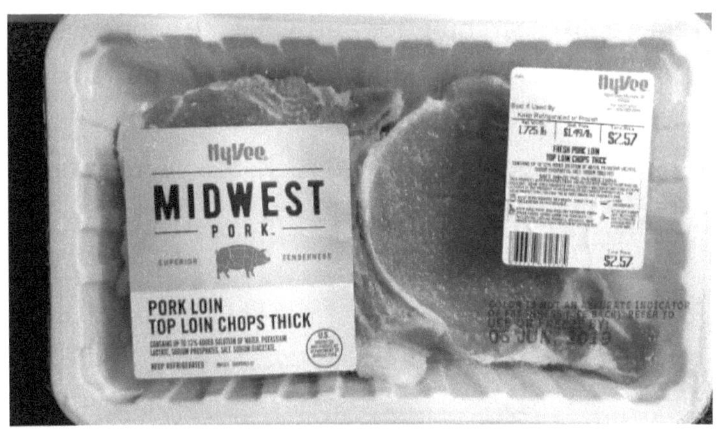

The websites flipp and MyGroceryDeals.com are recommended for you, the both of them will show sales in your area. You can also get some wonderful deals on steak in bulk by checking these sites often.

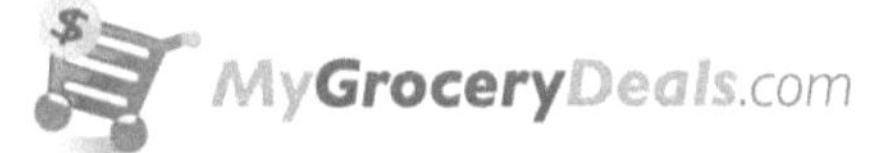

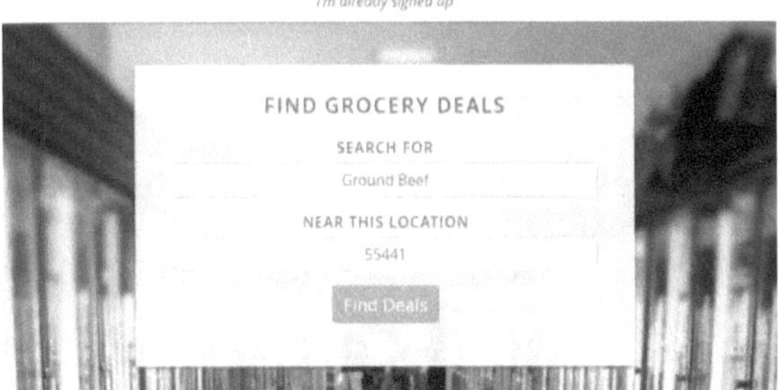

When you open the main page, it will ask you what item you're searching for and what ZIP code you're in.

What you need to do is—click the "Find Deals" button.

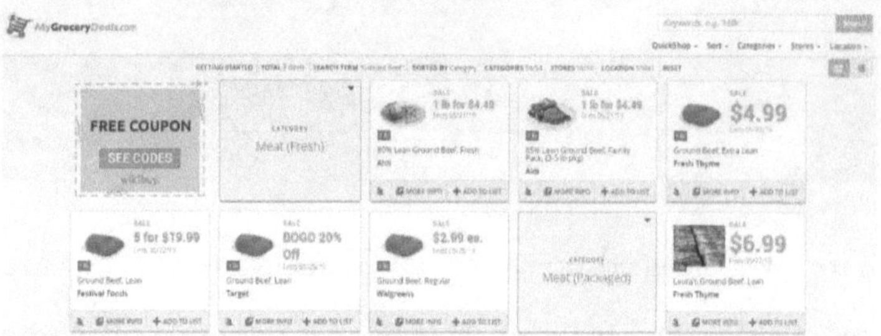

When you have clicked on the button, it will instantly return a result page that looks like the one above. It seems it searched out 16 nearby grocery stores and returned 7 deals for on-sale ground beef. #SWAG. So, you can visit this website often to get the lowest price of whatever you're searching for.

Most retailers have rewards programs or loyalty cards that are completely free and they provide certain discounts when scanned at the register. I recommend you sign up for all the ones that won't cost you anything. If you can get those exclusive deals that are reserved for only members, that will help you to save some cash!

Do not also forget wholesale stores! I recommend Costco for you as it is a great option.

Often and routinely, Costco and Sam's Club get praises from members of the carnivore and keto communities.

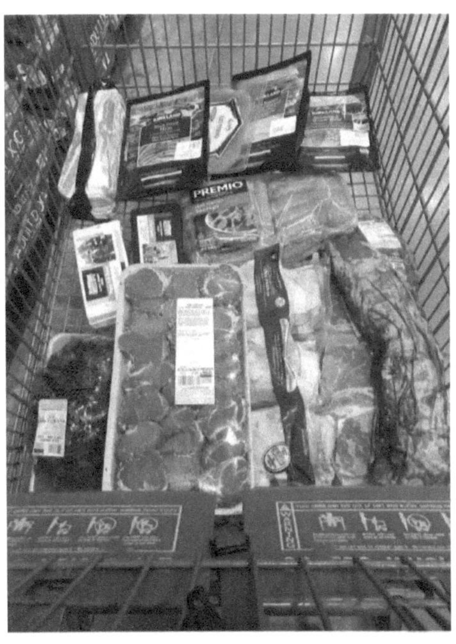

If your Costco cart doesn't always look like this, then know that you're doing it wrong.

Sadly, Costco steaks are blade-tenderized, that means that bacteria easily get pushed into the steak with needles, so I advise you to cook it until it is well-done (use 160 degrees) to be sure of your safety. But still, they have some very exciting deals that are not to be missed!

8. Eat lots of suet

You need to try out suet. It is very satiating and will help to cut down how much overall food you eat. Some people eat suet to satiation before they eat muscle meat, some believe it helps them to burn fat and to feel more satiated for the whole day.

Paradoxically, eating more fat can aid you to burn more fat.

Also, you can make friends with a local butcher and you would always get these trimmings free of charge or for about $1 or $2 a pound.

Suet is tasty and nutritious, and it is packed with a lot of fat-soluble vitamins.

Another great option for you is tallow. It can also help to add fats to your diet.

9. Find the Best Supermarket Deals

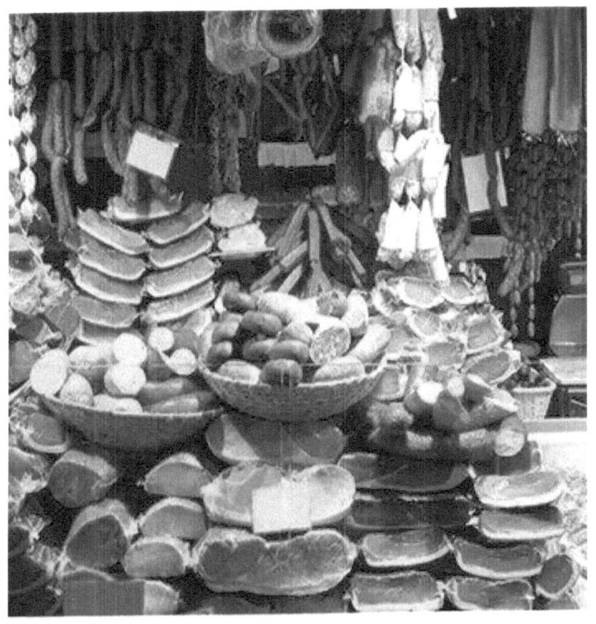

I try my best to stay away from big chain grocery store meat, as most of it is often highly processed. But then, if you're trying to engage in carnivore on a very low budget, then chain stores are the cheapest option for you.

If you always check out the websites for stores close to your home, then you can get any special meat deals they might be advertising. You might be lucky to see that they have good prices for your favorite ingredients!

For me though, I have found that my local butcher offers me great deals on a regular basis especially when I buy in bulk, and I trust his products more.

MEAT PRICE RANGES

To further help you get your fist carnivore diet prepared, I have listed some price ranges for different meats. With this, you can get an idea on how to maximize your calories per dollar spent.

1. Beef

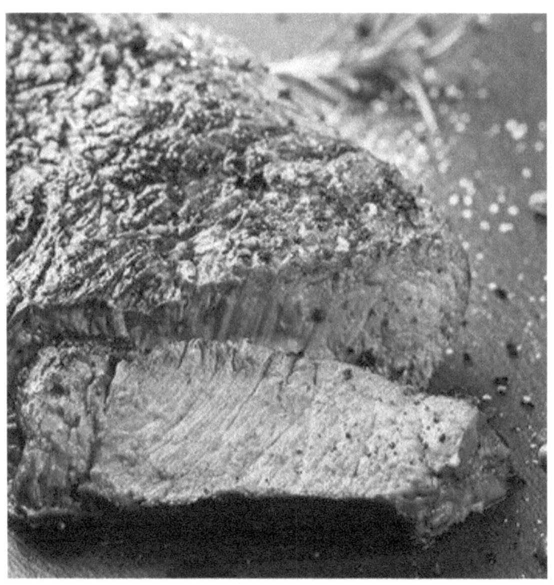

The cheapest in supermarkets are ground beef patties, but you must be careful to check if fillers are added as that could be introducing carbs. Less lean cuts (less than 70%) can be sold for about $3 per pound.

The price can be discounted if you buy in bulk and then freeze them.

For grass-fed rib-eye steaks, you'll get it for about $8, but you can reduce the cost by going for non-grass-fed options.

The good thing is ground beef is very versatile! You can use it to make meatballs burgers, or mix it with scrambled eggs. I love to make it into a burrito bowl using some bacon, sour cream and then top it with shredded cheese.

Just like eggs, tinned fish blends with beef especially as regards omega 3, vitamin D and Iodine. Make sure you buy these fish in water and not in oil.

2. Pork

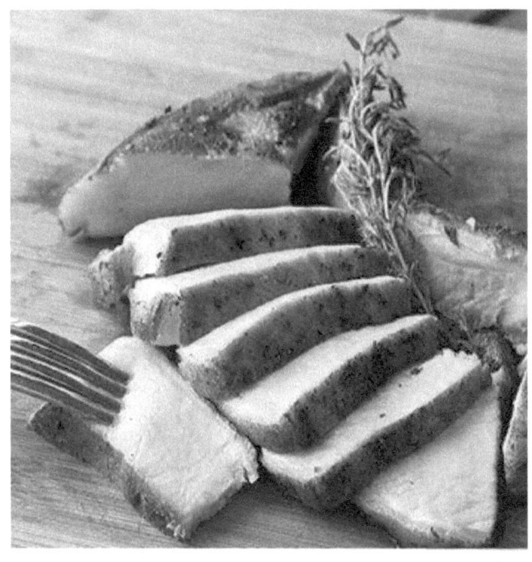

Pork belly is another great option for you. You can get it for as low as $2/lbs. It is very delicious especially when you prepare it well and slow cook it.

If you've had a poor experience with it, don't get turned off, as that is how the cooking method is.

Bacon and tenderloin cuts can be sold for about $6/lbs. They are very tasty and they can drive up your food costs.

3. Lamb

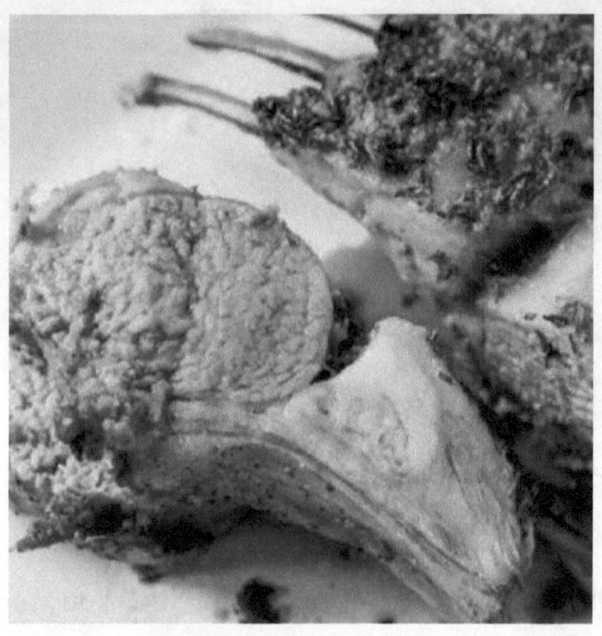

Sadly, you can't get "cheap" cuts of lamb like you can with pork and beef.

Nevertheless, you can buy lamb shanks for about $8/lbs., it depends on the time of year you are purchasing it.

I usually buy lamb as a treat, but if you want to reduce cost, then I advise you to go for other alternatives.

4. Chicken

You can get a high level of protein from chicken breasts and it cost about $3-3.5/lbs. or you can go for thighs as it is a considerably cheaper option. You can get thighs for about $2.5/lbs, the flavor on them are usually very good.

Some people love spicy wings, but they are actually not a good option for this diet, because you can't add the sauces.

Again, the meat on the wings is so little, so even though it's cheap, it doesn't profit you.

Check out Porter Road, there you can find whole chickens, one-in and boneless chicken breast and also fresh chicken broth for cooking.

5. Fish & Seafood

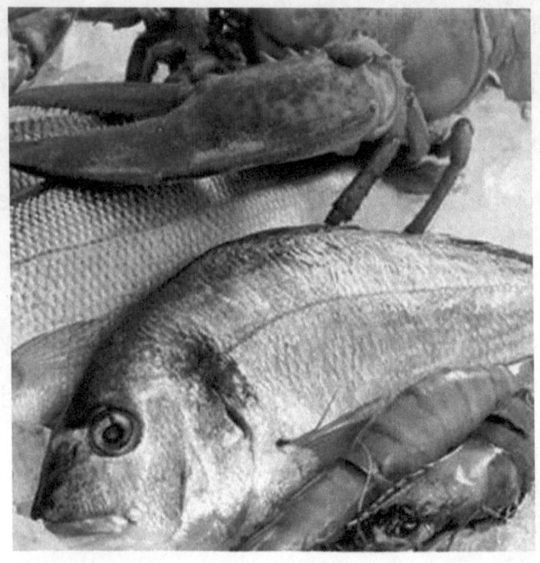

Fish can be quite expensive, especially if you go for cod and salmon.

Salmon can cost $10-12/lbs and cod around $6-8. However, they are excellent low-carb and high-fat food sources, they provide extra nutrients like vitamins, minerals, and fatty acids.

If you want the best go for mackerel. If you live close to the ocean, then go visit some fishing towns and see if you can buy some at wholesale prices of at least less than $2/lbs. Mackerel is filled with healthy fats and calories.

You can also get sardines, herring and anchovies. These cold-water, oily fish are nutrition powerhouses! A lot of carnivore promoters talk about eating nose-to-tail, that is, eating all organ meats and different parts of the animal. But if you are eating a sardine for example, you are eating the whole animal - right down to the bones!

6. Organ Meat

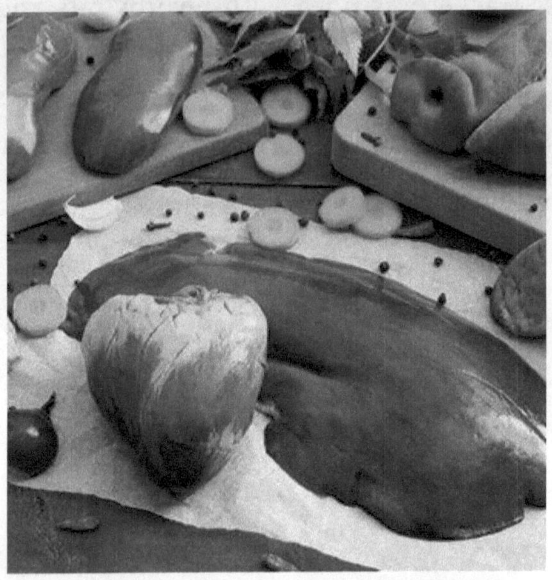

Liver, kidneys, and other organs are very rich in nutrients, most especially minerals, vitamins and animal protein.

I also advise you to consider bone marrow, you can buy it as a broth, and there are some that you can even buy that are organic and grass-fed, that's also not too expensive.

Most people are uncertain about it, but it's very sweet and nutritious.

Conclusion

Now you can see that there are various ways to reduce your food costs, though it may not be possible to live on $4 per day. If you are trying to lose weight on this diet, I suggest you eat eggs and cheese as they work as great fillers to keep you going.

You do not have any excuse to not try a carnivore diet for at least 30 days. It will make you see the issues that you didn't even know you had.

And in a lot of ways you can save money, especially if you major on reducing healthcare expenses for the rest of your life.

And if you are looking for extra convenience, you can try Butcher Box. They have constant promotions, and most times going yourself to get your groceries is not always worth the stress.

You can also engage in Intermittent fasting as it is a great way to lose weight and it will definitely help you to spend less on meat.